Summary

of

Norman Doidge's

The Brain That Changes Itself

Stories of Personal Triumph from the Frontiers of Brain Science

by
Swift Reads

Table of Contents

Overview

The Brain That Changes Itself: Stories of Personal Triumph from the Frontiers of Brain Science (2007) by psychiatrist Norman Doidge explores breakthroughs in neuroscience regarding plasticity, or the brain's ability to change. Doidge shares inspiring stories of the work done by what he calls "neuroplasticians"—neuroscientists who are pioneering new methods for optimizing brain function.

For four centuries, most scientists and doctors believed that brain anatomy was unchangeable; once the brain had developed post-childhood, it would not change again until beginning the age-related process of decline. In this view, patients who sustained brain injuries or other neurological damage were unfortunately doomed to a life of impairment and neurological dysfunction. The neurological decay associated with old age was also thought to be immovable and permanent.

These beliefs resulted from three factors. First, most people with brain injuries did appear to be permanently impaired. Second, for many years, scientists and doctors had no way of observing brain activities including the potential regeneration and reorganization of brain maps. Last, the belief that the brain was machine-like had been deeply ingrained since the dawn of modern science and therefore reinforced the notion of an unchangeable brain with fixed tasks assigned to particular local areas of the organ. In other words, the brain was hardwired, and this hardwiring was not subject to change.

Starting in the late 1960s and early 1970s, researchers began to make startling discoveries in the realm of neuroplasticity, learning that the brain is, in fact, changeable. The concept of plasticity was met with great resistance in the mainstream medical community. Yet the courage and curiosity of a handful of scientists brought plasticity to the fore, showing how plasticity can lead to flexible behaviors that increase adaptability and creativity, while improving functioning and quality of life. Over time, studies have revealed that the brain's structure can be strengthened or weakened, depending on the activities the brain engages in. For example, stroke patients who sustain damage to the areas of the brain that govern language and mobility can learn to speak and move again.

The brain is made up of neuronal pathways, or neurons that receive and transmit information to other neuronal cells. The human brain has approximately 100 billion neurons, and science is still in the process of uncovering the intricacies of neuronal function. When injury or disability disrupts neuronal pathways, the brain learns to use different pathways to perform the same function. Instinctively, the brain reorganizes itself. New experiences spark activity in different neurons; when these neurons are simultaneously activated, they release chemicals that bond them together, creating new neuronal pathways.

Previously, the brain was thought to be a separate entity from the mind, fixed and immovable. Understanding the ways in which mind and brain are inextricably linked allows for a more generous view of human potential.

Thanks to the ingenuity of some physicians and researchers, people who have experienced hearing or vision loss have regained function. Depression, anxiety, addiction, obsessive compulsive disorder, grief, and attachment issues can all be addressed and possibly alleviated through the prism of plasticity. Memory and cognitive functioning can be improved and strengthened into old age. Above all, neuroplasticity offers the hope that people, including those who face great adversities, can change and, perhaps most importantly, thrive.

Key Insights

1. Learning disabilities can be improved with specific brain exercises.

2. Brain development continues beyond the critical period of neurological development in childhood.

3. Brain maps are dynamic and plastic.

4. Pornography addictions are reflected in the brain by changed neuronal pathways.

5. Stroke patients who have lost language ability can be helped with constraint-induced (CI) therapies.

6. A plasticity-based approach is extremely helpful to those suffering with obsessive compulsive disorder (OCD).

7. Thoughts have the ability to alter brain structure.

8. In a phenomenon known as the "plastic paradox," the same neuroplastic characteristics that make flexibility possible also can lead to rigidity.

Key Insight 1

Learning disabilities can be improved with specific brain exercises.

Analysis

Conventional wisdom on treating learning disabilities has been to encourage compensations. For example, those with reading comprehension challenges might listen to audiobooks instead of reading. However, anecdotal evidence gathered by Barbara Arrowsmith Young, a Canadian educator, appears to show that students can at least partially recover from disabilities when they engage in exercises that heighten functioning in weakened brain areas, instead of avoiding those areas altogether.

In 2015, researchers at Stanford University published results of a study in *Nature Communications* on the role that neuroplasticity played in the academic success of students who had math-related learning disabilities. Learning disabled students who had one-on-one cognitive tutoring for eight weeks were found to have better comprehension of math problems. In addition to the improved performance, students registered changes in brain activity, particularly in the occipital areas associated with numerical problem solving. The improvements seemed greater than with behavioral interventions, such as compensations. While the researchers state that compensations can be helpful, cognitive tutoring for eight weeks appeared to bring the learning disabled students' brain activity up to the same level as that of their peers without learning disabilities—gains that do not occur with compensations or other behavioral methods. This study supports the notion that brain activity of learning disabled students can be improved to the level of their neurotypical peers with interventions that strengthen the weakened brain areas.

Key Insight 2

Brain development continues beyond the critical period of neurological development in childhood.

Analysis

Brain systems require prompts from external stimuli to develop. Each neural system of the brain has its own critical period when that system is more adaptable and capable of impressive growth. For example, the critical period for language starts when a baby is born and lasts through to approximately age 8. Previously, it was thought that growth could not occur after the critical periods ended, but recent breakthroughs in research have proven this theory wrong. The brain always has the potential to grow and regenerate.

In a 2017 article for *BBC Future,* writer David Robson shares inspiring examples of older people performing impressive feats—feats that support the idea of plasticity being accessible until death and counter the notion that the brain is fixed after its initial period of development. Robson highlights the achievements of Priscilla Sitienei, a 90-year-old midwife from Kenya who had never learned to read or write. Eager to record her knowledge for the next generation, Sitienei decided to go to school, learning in class alongside her great-great-grandchildren. In another example of plasticity at work beyond the critical period, Aleksandar Hemon found himself stuck in the US at the outbreak of the Bosnian war, unable to return to his home in Yugoslavia. Though Hemon had little fluency in English, his urgent need to write about the turmoil in his homeland was so great that he set out to learn English. Within three years, he published his first article in a journal. He went on to write several lauded literary books and to win the MacArthur Genius Award. Robson notes that staying physically fit seems to increase neuroplasticity. The act of learning a new activity also reminds older adults of the joys of learning and sparks a desire to engage in the world in fresh ways.

Key Insight 3

Brain maps are dynamic and plastic.

Analysis

The brain has different processing centers, which are called brain maps. Different maps are based in different regions. For example, motor maps, responsible for processing information that leads to movement, are located in the cerebral cortex. Contrary to what scientists initially thought, brain maps are changeable; they also vary in size and shape from person to person. With focused attention, brain maps can be redesigned to help people learn more efficiently and quickly, changing shape and size over the course of a lifetime.

In an example of dramatic advances in brain mapping, neurophysiologist Tony Zador of Cold Spring Harbor Laboratory in Long Island developed MAPseq, an innovative technology that can pinpoint specific neural pathways, highlighting tens of thousands of neural cells that have never before been seen. He spoke with *Quanta Magazine* in 2018 about the cutting-edge methodology and its implications for understanding brain functioning. In Zador's view, scientists don't know enough about neural circuitry, so he set out to change that. Looking at 50,000 neurons in the cerebral cortex of a mouse, Zador attributed a specific RNA code to each neuron. He then cut up the brain into cubes and inserted those cubes into a DNA sequencer, which enabled a 3D rendering of the mouse's cerebral cortex. Though MAPseq is still in development, Zador believes that it will one day be possible to use the same genomic sequencing method to account for the hundred billion neurons, as well as vast neural connections, in the brain. MAPseq opens the door to one day being able to look at and compare a variety of brains; understanding and measuring neural circuitry to this degree of detail will allow for the measurement of plasticity, showing exactly how different brain maps grow.

Key Insight 4

Pornography addictions are reflected in the brain by changed neuronal pathways.

Analysis

Some aspects of sexuality are subject to the brain's plasticity, such as the development of a pornography habit. With the rise of the Internet in the mid-nineties, pornography became more readily available—and more violent in nature. More people have become addicted to porn. As with other types of addictions, the brain becomes reliant on hits of dopamine, a feel-good neurotransmitter. Porn watching can unmask neural networks, a process by which existing neural networks that developed during the critical phase are strengthened. This unmasking process can reveal networks that were repressed in early childhood, during sexual development; watching porn joins these repressed networks with new neuronal pathways.

In 2011, researchers at the University of Texas at Austin took a comprehensive look at the scientific literature on excessive pornography use and the neurological changes that result; they also looked at various perspectives on pornography as a behavioral addiction. Addictions, including pornography addiction, lead to chemical alterations in the brain, as well as cerebral dysfunction. Brains damaged by addiction show lower activity in the frontal lobes, as has been extensively measured by magnetic resonance imaging (MRI) scans. This lower activity results in impulsivity, a disregard of the consequences of inappropriate behavior, and a lack of inhibition around inappropriate behavior. These changes are similar to those related to brain injuries. Dr. Howard Shaffer, a Harvard University psychiatrist, was one of the first to point out that addiction is the result of experience, and that neurocircuitry changes as a result of repetitive behaviors. Further, Shaffer believes there's little merit to debates on whether or not process addictions like pornography usage, which are behaviorally based, should be considered official addictions. His reasoning is based on the fact that behaviors like pornography usage spark the release of naturally generated chemicals; these neurotransmitters, according to Shaffer, are the "mediators" of addiction. Increasingly, it has become clear that while addictions may take different forms—such as alcohol, food, or pornography—the underlying structural changes of the brain are the same. Researchers at the University of Texas at Austin believe that embracing pornography addiction in neuroscientific terms will open up avenues of medical treatment, including with medication.

Key Insight 5

Stroke patients who have lost language ability can be helped with constraint-induced (CI) therapies.

Analysis

In addition to motor abilities, stroke patients often suffer loss of language, a condition also known as aphasia. Doctors have long thought that if recovery of language abilities hasn't been achieved within one year after a stroke, those abilities will not be recovered. This is not accurate, however. Many stroke patients show important gains from a form of CI therapy, in which patients are forced to use their language skills, however limited, to identify objects. It's possible for these gains to occur beyond the post-stroke year, and in some cases, years after the event.

For aphasia patients, recovering language skills can be arduous, which is why a speech rehabilitation group, run out of Touro College in Brooklyn, focuses on creating a happy atmosphere, as chronicled in a 2015 *Quartz* article. Staying upbeat is especially important for members of Professor Isabella Reichel's group, who have an added layer of difficulty: they're non-native

English speakers. As Russian immigrants, the members of Reichel's group have a better chance of relearning lost language skills in their native language. Not only can Reichel, who was born and raised in the Ukraine, offer these aphasia patients exercises in Russian, but she shares many cultural referents. Activities revolve around singing Russian folk songs and bringing in pictures from home that will jog memories and spark conversation. Izy, an older member who has recovered his language skills, still comes faithfully, using humor to try to help others speak. The main obstacles, according to Reichel, are for the patients to find the words they want to use, formulate sentences, and have the courage to speak. The social bonds between group members, including Reichel, help to give these aphasia patients the added push they need to persevere. Reichel is insistent that members push themselves to find and use words, even when it is difficult, and the care she exhibits for all the members encourages them to try, even when trying feels impossible. Reichel's focus on positivity is intentional—and science-based. She explains that when people feel good, their left frontal lobes generate dopamine, which makes it easier to process information. Reichel's methodology is a form of CI therapy—she is firm that the stroke patients exercise language skills. Her example of creating a buoyant atmosphere proves that CI therapy and stroke and language recovery can at times be uplifting.

Key Insight 6

A plasticity-based approach is extremely helpful to those suffering with obsessive compulsive disorder (OCD).

Analysis

OCD behaviors, such as obsessive hand-washing, become wired into the brain. An effective way to break up the negative wiring is to have those with OCD shift their focus away from obsessive thoughts to something else, like listening to a podcast or admiring the colors of the sky. Over time, this change of attention breaks neural pathways that have been strengthened by giving in to compulsions.

Take the hypothetical example of Andrea, a middle-aged mother whose eight-year-old child has a grave disease. In response to her grief, Andrea has developed some tics. For example, she cannot leave the house without checking, double checking, and triple checking all the lights in the house are off. She worries that while she is out, the house will burn down. Even after incessant checking of all fire hazards, Andrea still ruminates when she's not at home. At medical appointments and other errands, Andrea's mind will drift to images of coming home to fire trucks in front of her house. If her husband is home, she will call or text him and ask him to check all the lights in the house and to make sure the iron is unplugged. He quickly becomes tired of her anxiety; they have enough to cope with as a family, without Andrea's fixation. At the urging of her husband, she goes to see a therapist who gives her a simple protocol; when her mind starts racing, she is to take a deep breath and take note of physical details around her—the color of her sofa, for example, or the sound and quality of her daughter's voice. Once she is grounded in the present moment, Andrea can detach from her fears by recognizing that they are not reality-based. From there, she can consciously change her thoughts to focus on something more positive, such as gratitude. This habit eventually becomes wired into the brain. So, every time she doesn't give into obsessive thinking, she strengthens neural pathways that support a calm, centered mind, while breaking the neural pathways that support her obsessive compulsive thinking. In effect, her meditative practices have molded her habit of obsessive thinking out of her brain.

Key Insight 7

Thoughts have the ability to alter brain structure.

Analysis

Research has shown that the ways that people think can shape brain activity and structure. For example, in one study, researchers compared the brain activity of two groups: one that played a sequence on the piano and one that only imagined playing the sequence. At the end of the study, both groups showed the same brain changes—the region responsible for motor signals had grown. This study, along with others, proves that what people think impacts brain activity.

The mind-body connection has surprising implications for overall health, too, as social scientist Ellen Langer explores in *Counter Clockwise: Mindful Health and the Power of Possibility* (2009). Over the course of her career, Langer has explored how the mind affects physical health. Her 2010 study done at Harvard University illustrated just how powerful the mind can be. One group of housekeepers was told that exercising didn't need to be arduous and that their daily activities at work met Centers for Disease Control

(CDC) exercise requirements. The researchers even shared information about how many calories were burned in specific instances, such as changing linens. The second group of housekeepers was not given this information about exercise. At the end of four weeks, subjects in the former group had lost weight and body mass, even though *neither group's behavior had changed.* The power of suggestion—perhaps a bit of placebo, the mere belief that their daily work would contribute to heightened health—had been enough to create physical changes. A person's mindset is intricately linked to brain function and as a result, overall health and well being.

Key Insight 8

In a phenomenon known as the "plastic paradox," the same neuroplastic characteristics that make flexibility possible also can lead to rigidity.

Analysis

The "plastic paradox" dictates that the same mechanisms by which the brain can change allow for the brain to become rigid as well. Consider the metaphor of a sled going down a snow-covered hill. The first time, the sled creates a new pathway through fresh snowfall. But if the sled goes down that same pathway two or three more times, the path becomes deeper, making the forging of a new pathway unlikely. It is the same with neural pathways. Any type of consistent repetition that occurs without variation can lead to rigid behaviors.

Because neural pathways formed in childhood impact adult functioning, it's imperative that parents understand how to best support brain adaptability in their children, as physician Daniel J. Siegel and psychotherapist Tina Bryson explore in *No Drama Discipline: The Whole Brain Way to Calm the Chaos and Nurture Your Child's*

Developing Mind (2014). To best encourage flexibility and healthy brain development—the opposite of rigidity—Siegel and Bryson suggest that parents adopt a healthy attitude toward challenging experiences. Even boredom, when viewed through the right lens, is an opportunity for a growing child's brain to learn about flexibility and creativity. So parents should not step in when children complain of being bored. Parents can also help to guide children who have faced or are facing tough experiences. Instead of trying to shield them completely, parents can help children understand that adversity is always an opportunity to learn something important about themselves and the world. This will lessen the child's association with problems as traumas and encourage resiliency; with this approach, children learn to accept and face problems directly, without catastrophizing. This is one way that parents can plant seeds for plasticity that can make children less likely to get stuck in negative neural pathways.

Important People

Norman Doidge is a Canadian psychiatrist and bestselling author. He teaches in the Department of Psychiatry at the University of Toronto and Columbia University's Center for Psychoanalytic Training and Research.

Barbara Arrowsmith Young is an educator, child development specialist, and founder of the Arrowsmith School for children with learning disabilities.

Author's Style

Norman Doidge writes with great enthusiasm about breakthroughs in neuroscience, particularly in the realm of neuroplasticity, or the brain's ability to change itself. In each chapter, he brings research areas and concepts to life via the personal experiences of doctors, researchers, and patients whose lives best illustrate these principles. He also shares stories of difficulties that pioneers of plasticity have had to face, such as colleagues who disapprove of the concept, as it's a departure from mainstream medical knowledge. The genuine appreciation and admiration he has for neuroplasticians is evident throughout the book. The book is divided into 11 chapters, covering plasticity as it relates to a range of topics, including love and sex, grief, the imagination, addictions, and psychoanalysis. Each chapter includes a story of triumph, such as that of Michelle Mack, a woman whose left hemisphere never developed; her right hemisphere rewired itself so that it could perform brain functions of the missing hemisphere. In addition to the preface and index, there's an extensive listing of notes, some of which are academic and some of which provide further material to contemplate. There are also two appendices, one on culture and one on progress.

Readers may find some of Doidge's ideas somewhat off-putting, such as his thoughts on sexuality; what some readers consider to be normal forms of sexual expression, such as bondage, Doidge reduces to pathologies, adhering closely to Freudian ideas about sexual repression. His descriptions of experiments on animals, including kittens, may also disturb readers. He writes glowingly of the scientists and doctors he includes in this book, though some of the work he highlights has been controversial. For example, Barbara Arrowsmith Young has been criticized for claims she makes about her method to cure learning disabilities. Detractors say that she hasn't tested her claims in independent, peer-reviewed studies. Early on, Doidge sets up the idea that neuroplasticians have had to buck tradition and risk disapproval and ridicule of their peers, so it's easy to imagine why he doesn't present Arrowsmith Young's ideas with a critical eye.

Author's Perspective

Doidge is a well-respected researcher, practitioner, and educator. After completing his psychiatric and psychoanalytic training at Columbia University's Department of Psychiatry, Doidge was a Columbia-National Institute of Health Fellow for two years and a Clinical Fellow in Psychiatry at Columbia University. He has received many awards for his scientific contributions in psychiatry and psychoanalysis.

In addition to his scientific pursuits, he is a successful author. *The Brain That Changes Itself* has sold more than one million copies. *The Brain's Way of Healing*, his second book, was awarded the Gold Nautilus Award in Science in 2015. Prior to becoming an author, he was an award-winning magazine writer, with an eye for human interest stories.

Manufactured by Amazon.ca
Bolton, ON

17895802R00017